THE NURSING ASSISTANT'S SURVIVAL GUIDE

Second Edition

Tips & Techniques for the Most
Important Job in America

Karl Pillemer, Ph.D

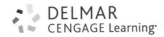

DELMAR
CENGAGE Learning

Australia • Brazil • Japan • Korea • Mexico • Singapore • Spain • United Kingdom • United States

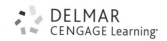

The Nursing Assistant's Survival Guide, Second Edition
Karl Pillemer

Vice President, Career and Computing: Dave Garza

Director of Learning Solutions: Matthew Kane

Senior Acquisitions Editor: Maureen Rosener

Managing Editor: Marah Bellegarde

Product Manager: Samantha L. Miller

Vice President, Career and Professional Marketing: Jennifer Ann Baker

Marketing Director: Wendy E. Mapstone

Senior Marketing Manager: Michele McTighe

Marketing Coordinator: Scott A. Chrysler

Senior Production Director: Wendy Troeger

Production Manager: Andrew Crouth

Content Project Management: PreMediaGlobal

Senior Art Director: Jack Pendleton

Cover image: Courtesy of iStock.com

For product information and technology assistance, contact us at **Cengage Learning Customer & Sales Support, 1-800-354-9706**

For permission to use material from this text or product, submit all requests online at **www.cengage.com/permissions.** Further permissions questions can be e-mailed to **permissionrequest@cengage.com**

Library of Congress Control Number: 2012933445

ISBN-13: 978-1-133-13481-7

ISBN-10: 1-133-13481-5

Delmar
5 Maxwell Drive
Clifton Park, NY12065-2919
USA

Cengage Learning is a leading provider of customized learning solutions with office locations around the globe, including Singapore, the United Kingdom, Australia, Mexico, Brazil, and Japan. Locate your local office at: **international.cengage.com/region**

Cengage Learning products are represented in Canada by Nelson Education, Ltd.

To learn more about Delmar, visit www.**cengage.com/delmar**

Purchase any of our products at your local college store or at our preferred online store www.**cengagebrain.com**

Printed in the United States of America
1 2 3 4 5 6 7 16 15 14 13 12

Contents

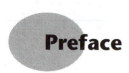
Preface

Introduction

This new edition of the *Nursing Assistant's Survival Guide* is filled with concrete tips designed to develop and hone the interpersonal skills needed for job success. Thoroughly updated to reflect recent changes in the field, this handy guide includes step-by-step information about how to handle specific problems such as managing job stress, dealing with death on the job, being a good communicator, getting along with your supervisor, relating to family members, working with aggressive residents, and balancing work and family.

To the CNA

There are many reasons I wrote this book, but the biggest one is that I think you have one of the most important jobs in the world. There really isn't a more worthwhile profession than to work hands-on, one-on-one, with someone in the last stages of life. It is a noble mission to care for older people.

Long experience has taught us that CNAs need two kinds of knowledge to become truly successful at their jobs. One kind of knowledge you already have: the technical skills to be able to do your job. You've learned about things like how to bathe and feed residents, transfer procedures, infection control, and residents' rights.

But this is only one part of the job—and not the hardest part! What's hardest for most CNAs is handling the interpersonal and emotional aspects of the job. As the interpersonal side includes working with family members, helping residents who have behavior problems, grieving for residents who die, working with a supervisor, managing time wisely, and reducing stress, the CNA's job is very, very complicated. To succeed, you need to expand your skills as a "people person." That's where this guide will be useful.

Organization and How to Use this Guide

How should you use this book?

This book will help you approach your work situation with your eyes wide open. I'm not going to cover up the difficult aspects of being a CNA, but I'm going to try to help you enjoy and appreciate the rewarding parts of your job and to survive the hard parts.

I'll give you the inside information that will help you get the most out of being a CNA. These suggestions are based on what my colleagues and I have seen most long-term CNAs go through.

If you are new to CNA work, then I would like to help you get off to the right start. If you are an experienced CNA, this guide can provide you with new skills and ideas to improve your work life.

The Development Process

Over the years, I've learned about what many CNAs believe are the hardest parts of the job. These are the kinds of situations where you ask *What do I do now?* I've taken eight of those truly difficult issues and found some answers for you. I've talked to well-known experts, and I've talked to plenty of CNAs (who are experts, too!).

Each of the chapters takes you through a single problem and helps you to see it in a new way. You'll get step-by-step guidance about how to handle the situation. You'll read advice from other CNAs and you'll learn that you're not alone in struggling with that problem—lots of other people are trying to solve it, too.

These are the issues this book will help you address:

- Handling job stress
- Dealing with the death of residents
- Being a good communicator
- Getting along with your supervisor
- Relating to family members
- Working with angry and aggressive residents
- Balancing work and family
- Maintaining a positive attitude

You don't have to sit down and read this book from cover to cover. Some people will want to do this (they are the ones who have to eat their vegetables before they can have dessert!), but others may just want to go to the chapters that interest them the most. After you've read it, you may want to refer back to the book from time to time for a fresh look at these issues.

No one knows what to do in every situation that comes up in a nursing home, but in the chapters that follow, we've gathered the best advice available. We think you will find it useful and encouraging.

New to this Edition

The second edition includes a new chapter that describes the use of positive psychology and humor in daily practice, along with other powerful tools to reduce stress and lift your spirits.

New material on handling work/life conflicts has been added, as well as sections specifically addressing person-centered care. Each of the topics found here has been thoroughly updated to reflect recent developments in the CNA field.

Acknowledgments

This book is dedicated to those who do the hardest, most important job in America—nursing assistants. Were it not for their commitment, compassion, and skill, our elders would be without the loving care they deserve. Angels of mercy, guardians, healers, heroes—they are a shining example to us all.

Reviewers

Anna Ortigara, RN, MS, FAAN
Director of Communication and Outreach,
THE GREEN HOUSE Project
Tinley Park, Illinois

Genevieve Gipson
Director, National Network of Career Nursing Assistants
Norton, Ohio

About the Author

Karl Pillemer

Karl Pillemer, PhD, is a Professor in the Human Development Department at Cornell University and Director of the Cornell Institute for Translational Research on Aging. Throughout his career, Dr. Pillemer has conducted research and developed practical programs to improve the work life of nursing home staff. He is also a founder and consulting editor of *Nursing Assistant Monthly*, a newsletter that reaches thousands of certified nursing assistants each month.

What do I do when . . .

There's too much stress?

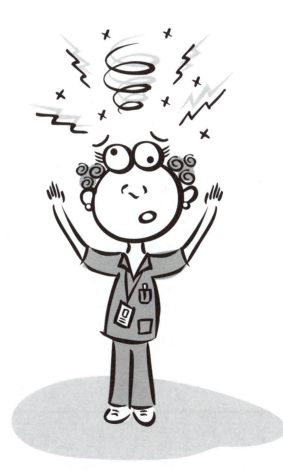

Nursing assistants have a stressful job. In surveys, over two-thirds of nursing home staff report feeling stressed and burned out at least some of the time. Fortunately, stress doesn't have to ruin your work life. The better you understand the causes and effects of stress, the easier it is to manage daily hassles and make your job easier.

1st The first thing to do:
Understand CNA stress

Sandy's day got off to a bad start. Her four-year-old woke up with a bad cold and couldn't go to day care. She arranged a babysitter, but then she had trouble starting her car. When she arrived at work 15 minutes late, she learned that one of the other nursing assistants had called in sick. Since her facility couldn't find a replacement, they would be "working short" that day.

As she began work, Sandy became worried about the rest of the day. *How will I get everything done,* she asked herself, *especially when we're down a person?* She felt her heart begin to beat harder, her stomach tighten, and her breathing get faster. *Maybe I'm the one who needs to call in sick,* she thought.

Sandy is feeling the symptoms of stress. All of us feel this way from time to time on our jobs. It is the sense of being overwhelmed by all that we have to do, and of having deadlines that are hard to meet. And problems at home just add to our stress level at work.

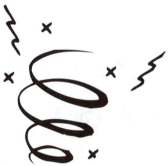

© Delmar/Cengage Learning 2013

What is stress?

Stress occurs when we feel a threat to our well-being and we aren't sure how to deal with it. You can imagine what happens when there is a physical threat, for example, if a large, angry dog begins to chase you. Your body automatically acts by either preparing to fight the threat or to run away from it.

Your body does the same thing even when the threat isn't right there for you to see. When work gets to be too much, our bodies respond in a big way: muscles get tense, digestion slows down, blood sugar rises, heart rate quickens, and breathing gets faster (sound familiar?).

When stress occurs a lot, we can start to have emotional and physical problems. Some signs of too much stress are the following:

- Feeling like you can't slow down or relax
  - Getting really angry over small things
    - Being anxious or tense for more than a few days
      - Having trouble paying attention to things
      - Feeling extremely tired
    - Having physical symptoms such as not sleeping well or tension headaches
- Using alcohol or medications more often

© Delmar/Cengage Learning 2013

No matter how much you want to help others, and no matter how hard you try to stay cheerful, there are some days when being a nursing assistant can make you feel empty and blue. A good way to describe these feelings is the term *burnout*. When we say we're "burned out," we mean feeling overwhelmed, stressed, or unhappy because of our work.

Stress and burnout are very important problems for CNAs. In our surveys, about 70% of CNAs say they feel burned out some of the time. They say that they feel like they often can't do all their assigned tasks. The stress of working when there are not enough staff on the unit also causes burnout. CNAs tell us that problems with their supervisors, other CNAs, family members, and residents are all sources of stress and burnout.

Besides these kinds of problems, stress also causes trouble for your nursing home. Why? Because the greater the stress and burnout, the more likely CNAs are to leave their jobs. And people who are burned out have less to give to the residents.

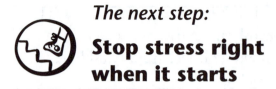

The next step:

Stop stress right when it starts

When you start to feel stressed, you need to have something you can do. Here are three things you can do right when you begin to feel stressed. All three of these activities have been shown to reduce stress. Try each one of them, and see which works best for you.

To relax, breathe deeply

Stress causes your breathing to become shallow, making you feel more stressed. To avoid this problem, take time when you're feeling stressed to breathe deeply. You will soon feel calm again. Breathe in through your nose while you slowly count from one to five. Release the breath at the same slow pace, counting backward from five to one. Repeat this a few times—In: 1, 2, 3, 4, 5; Out: 5, 4, 3, 2, 1.

To relax, tense up!

Tensing and then relaxing muscles can be a good way to relax. Take a few minutes to try this exercise: Start by squinting your eyes and clenching your teeth. Release them after three to four seconds and feel the warmth as the tension disappears. Repeat this procedure by hunching your shoulders and tensing your stomach muscles. Again, after a few seconds, release and feel the difference. Now try tensing your hands and arms—and again, release to feel the change.

© Delmar/Cengage Learning 2013

Finally, tense up your legs and toes. When you let go, become aware of the calm, relaxed feeling in your whole body.*

Think your stress away

Boston physician and researcher Dr. Herbert Benson is one of the leading experts on stress reduction. He suggests that a way to reduce stress is through "mindfulness." By this he means focusing your attention on what you are experiencing in a given moment. You become aware of your own feelings and what's going on around you. This helps you slow your thoughts down, and helps bring about what Benson calls the "relaxation response."

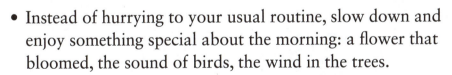

© Delmar/Cengage Learning 2013

Taken directly from his book, *The Wellness Book,*** here are some of his suggestions for using mindfulness to relax in your workday:

- Instead of hurrying to your usual routine, slow down and enjoy something special about the morning: a flower that bloomed, the sound of birds, the wind in the trees.

- When stopped at a traffic light or waiting for the bus, check your body for signs of physical tension. Drop your shoulders, release your hands on the wheel, soften your facial muscles. Can you break the cycle of running yellow lights and passing cars?

- When you arrive at your workplace, take a few moments to orient yourself, breathe consciously and calmly, and relax your body; then begin.

- When at work, become aware of the signs of physical tension. Take some mindful breaths to relax and release tension.

- As you return home, can you consciously make the transition from work to home? If possible, after greeting your family or housemates, give yourself a few minutes alone to ease the transition.

- As you go to sleep, let go of today and tomorrow, and take some slow, mindful breaths.

(?) *What else can I do?*
Consider some lifestyle changes

If you try the activities listed above, you will be able to calm yourself at work even when things seem out of control. But you also need to see if some things in your life can be changed to make you less likely to get stressed in the first place. Think about these:

Take a look at your lifestyle

Changing certain habits will lower stress. Cutting down on caffeine, for example, may relieve anxiety and the jitters. Getting eight hours of sleep will ensure that you function at your best. And exercising for 30 minutes, three to four times per week, can greatly reduce your stress levels and improve your feeling of well-being. This doesn't mean a trip to the gym. You can get some walking in just by parking your car farther away from work. You can put on an aerobics tape at home or just climb the stairs a few times in your apartment building. Getting exercise will make you feel better when you are at work.

Look for social support

Social support is a major stress reducer. When you are down, you need friends to turn to, especially in a long-term care facility. Talk about problems that are causing you stress. Share solutions with others.

Look for positive people who seem to be coping well with the stress and strain of the work. Although we all complain sometimes, avoid coworkers who are always whining. It may make them feel better to do so (but probably not), but it certainly won't help you to bounce back from feeling low. The answer to discouragement is encouragement: Find coworkers who will lift your spirits and remember to do the same for them when they're feeling bad.

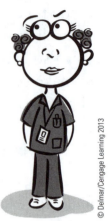

© Delmar/Cengage Learning 2013

Seek professional help if you need it

Stress can get the best of anybody. If your stress-related symptoms just won't go away, you might want to consult a counselor. If your facility has an employee assistance program (EAP), you can begin there. Otherwise, a social worker or personal physician will serve as a good resource. Trained professionals can help you learn to manage stress and to improve the quality of your life.

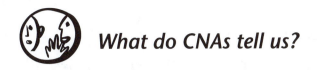 *What do CNAs tell us?*

Here's how some CNAs responded to the question:

What do you do when you feel stressed?

JUANITA FERGUSON

Mark Rest Center, McConnelsville, Ohio

"I get a little bit silly with the other nurse aides. We joke around. I try to make light of the situation."

PAT WESTON

El Carino TCU, Santa Fe, New Mexico

"I'll talk to someone, whether it be a supervisor, the administrator, or another aide. With a difficult patient I might ask another aide how they have handled the patient in the past. Or if another aide is able to deal with the patient a little better I'll ask her to switch with me and I'll care for one of hers. I come to work with the attitude that there are certain things that I have to do, and I go about my business."

EDNA FULLENWINDER

Inman Health Care, Inman, South Carolina

"I'll go and talk with some residents—some of them can tell a good joke. They make me feel better and forget that it's raining. Some of them remember my name, my children's names, my husband's name, my mama's name. They want to talk about it."

JOYCE COLEMAN

Preakness Hospital, Haledon, New Jersey

"We have peer group meetings once a month that are chaired by our floor social worker. No supervisors are present, so you can say whatever you have to say. We use these meetings to get out our frustrations."

CHERYL KNIGHT

Parkview, Paducah, Kentucky

"We have a great charge nurse, so I take things up with her. She always seems to know the right things to say and do, even if it's just a hug."

Remember

- **Get enough sleep.**

- **Avoid too much caffeine.**

- **Exercise regularly.**

- **Talk to other people about problems on the job.**

- **Talk to a counselor or physician if you are feeling very stressed.**

- **Use deep breathing and relaxation on the job to feel less stressed.**

Sources:

* *The Doctors' Guide to Instant Stress Relief;* Ronald G. Nathan, Thomas E. Staats, and Paul J. Roschand; Ballantine Books, 1989.

* *The Wellness Book;* Herbert Benson and Eileen M. Stuart; Simon and Schuster, 1992; pages 56–57.

What do I do when . . .

A resident dies?

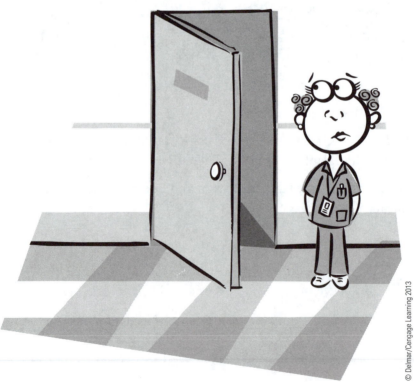

Unfortunately, the death of residents happens all the time in the nursing home. This can make you feel upset, stressed, and burned out. Many CNAs find it hard to deal with the sadness they feel after a resident they were close to dies.

People might think that CNAs just get used to residents dying. However, experts have found that nursing assistants are often seriously affected by the death of residents. CNAs are the ones who make life go on in a nursing home after a resident dies. But it is important that they take the time to mourn the death of residents who were especially close to them.

The first thing to do:

1st Understand and accept grieving

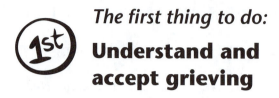

QUESTION: **What do the following symptoms have in common?**

tightness in the throat • weakness • shortness of breath • the need to sigh • an empty feeling • weakness • crying • fainting • abnormal sweating

ANSWER: **They can all be the natural results of bereavement.**

All of the bereavement symptoms listed above are parts of a process called grief. And no matter how used you get to the fact that your residents die, you will feel some grief when you lose a favorite resident. If you're an experienced CNA, you've probably felt grief more than once. But, like many people, you may not have known how to handle it. The death of residents, and the need to grieve, is a major source of stress and burnout for CNAs.

© Delmar/Cengage Learning 2013

Grief is a natural and normal process. In fact, many experts believe that allowing ourselves to feel grief actually helps us recover from a death. Unfortunately, in nursing home work, it is not always easy to go through the grieving process.

Grief over a death has physical symptoms. Sometimes, a grieving person can't eat, sleep, or perform many of his or her daily activities. The problem is made harder for nursing assistants, who often are not given the time to grieve and instead have to move along with the demands of their work.

What is "grief"?

Many experts suggest that grieving people often share several common experiences:

- The most common responses to death are feelings of shock, numbness, and disbelief that the person has actually died.

- Soon, the shock and disbelief usually give way to wanting to have the dead person back again. During this period, it is natural for grieving people to intensely miss the dead person. People sometimes think they hear the dead person's voice or even see an illusion of him or her. Other feelings can include guilt, irritability, restlessness, or many of these and other feelings at the same time.

- People can get depressed or anxious while they are grieving.

- Finally, the good news is this: You will recover from grief. After recovering, people can see themselves in a new light, and they often feel like they have learned something from the experience.

With your residents, you may not experience all of these symptoms, or you may only experience them mildly. But we've heard many nursing assistants say something like this: "What?! Mrs. S died? How can that be? I was just chatting with her yesterday, and she seemed fine!" The point is, you need to allow yourself to feel these emotions if they arise.

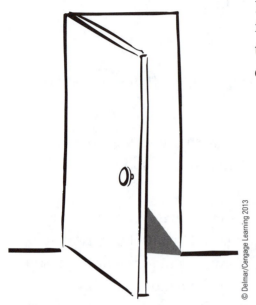

© Delmar/Cengage Learning 2013

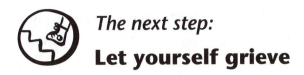

The next step:

Let yourself grieve

Follow your own pace

Nursing assistants should remember that everyone grieves in his or her own way and at his or her own pace. Grieving is never easy, but it is normal. No one can take away the pain that is felt during bereavement. However, it helps to know what to expect from grief (for example, that it's normal to be sad). And talking with friends and family about how you feel can also help.

Death and dying expert Franne Whitney Nelson gives this advice:

> *Because of the long-term nature of most nursing home stays, nursing assistants can expect to become attached to many of their residents. In fact, some residents may become as well-loved by the nursing assistant as the nursing assistant's own family members. Therefore, when a resident dies, it can be the same as if a family member died. We're always affected when someone dies. If we don't cry, the unshed tears build up and this can have many negative effects, both psychological and physical. Nursing assistants must give themselves permission to feel their feelings. They must shed the tears that come naturally. There are no nobler tears than those shed for others. Not crying encourages others to do the same, when nursing assistants should really be trying to do their part to create an environment in which death is not shameful.*

So we'll be honest with you. When you work in a nursing home, you see up close a fact of life that we often prefer not to think about: People get old, and sick, and they die. As a CNA, you have to learn how to deal with the sadness you feel. Some nursing homes conduct a service for residents who die in the facility. Try to attend these services, especially if you were close to the resident. Being part of a service or ceremony can help you feel supported in your grief.

Remember, grief is real and natural. The key to helping other CNAs deal with grief is to be patient and understand that grief is something we all share. One day you will need the support of others, too. Your compassion and generosity toward a grieving coworker can begin to create an environment in which the death and grief that are an unavoidable part of working in a nursing home can be talked about openly and honestly.

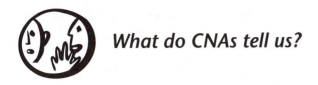 ## What do CNAs tell us?

Many career CNAs tell us that caring for the dying is one of the most rewarding aspects of their job. We interviewed two CNAs who have thought a lot about this issue: Marie Welch and Edward Diggins of Mariner Health Care of Merrimack Valley, Amesbury, Massachusetts. Here's what they had to say:

What was your first experience with death on the job?

Marie: *I was scared. I was brand new and within the first hours on the job, someone died. It left me with the impression that if I was going to see someone die, I needed someone with me. It's very different from a family member passing away; this is a whole different ball game.*

Edward: *Actually, it was three weeks ago. I have only been here six months so that was my first experience. Her name was Annie and her quality of life at that point wasn't so good. It was no surprise; I was expecting it. It left me with mild sadness because CNAs get used to taking care of someone, and then they aren't there anymore. That's how I felt the loss. Personalities are gone—you notice they aren't there anymore.*

Have you ever had to prepare the body of a resident who just died? And if so, how did you get through it?

Marie: *Yes, that very first day. That's why I was so scared. Getting through it . . . now I talk to the body like the person is still alive. I tell them, "Okay, I'm rolling you over now." I'm used to taking care of people when they are alive in this way, so I continue after they die.*

What's the hardest thing for you in coping with the death of residents?

Edward: *Watching their families struggling with the loss. I want to be supportive, but I'm not feeling my best either. So I put others' needs before my own. That's my job, and that's what I focus on.*

Marie: *Like Edward said, it's seeing the families. You take care of them, speak with them honestly and make them comfortable. You tell yourself to wait until you get home.*

How does your family react?

Marie: *They understand. They know it's part of the job.*

What determines whether a CNA stays in this career? What is it about a person that allows one to deal with death?

Edward: *For some people, the sadness is too overwhelming. They get attached to a person and they don't know how to unattach themselves. Sometimes they get tired of bringing home the sadness to their families. It's a life choice they have to make. Nursing assistants are expected to do physical work and emotional work at the same time. When CNAs separate the two, or don't balance them, that's when they leave. Denial doesn't work here.*

Marie: *Death sometimes stresses people out so bad, they run from it. They don't want to think about it or deal with it. If you want to be a CNA, you have to have a strong stomach, a good will, and a good heart. You have to know how to joke too. This work isn't for everyone.*

What would your advice be to new nursing assistants adjusting to this type of environment?

Marie: *I would suggest that supervisors and other CNAs don't throw new ones into situations like I was when I first began. Just begin by asking if they want to be in the room when the body is prepared and washed. Let them watch and ask questions. Just don't jump into it.*

Edward: *I agree . . . take things slowly. You've chosen this work so you shouldn't be surprised; nonetheless, you need to prepare. Before starting the job, look at your own experience of death with maybe your own relatives, and then use your feelings as a guide. And balance attachments. Always remember that the residents are dependent on you; you are not dependent on them. Keeping that in mind lightens the load. If you do your job right, the resident has had comfortable last days and that should make you feel good about your work.*

How do nursing assistants help each other out during these times of loss?

Edward: *We talk a lot and get it all out. In this job, you talk all the time anyway, about the patient's progress, about the families, about what needs to be done. Death and coping in the nursing home is a gradual arc, not a sudden jolt. It's a shared experience, common to us all. We are not on our own here, and we discuss our feelings, our moods. It's almost like having a therapist around because emotions aren't hanging around inside you—it's no secret and little by little, the feelings get worked out.*

Remember

When a resident dies, be sure to

• **let yourself grieve.**

• **ask for help from other staff.**

• **offer support to other grieving staff.**

• **offer support to the resident's family.**

What do I do when . . .

I have trouble communicating?

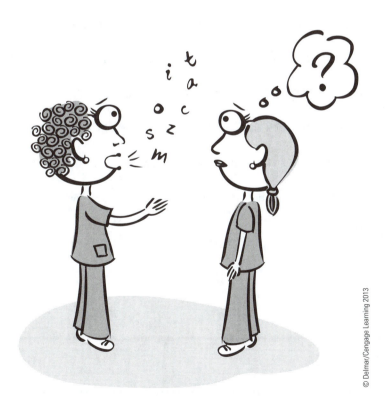

TIDEWATER COMMUNITY COLLEGE

The best CNAs are also good communicators. They have to be! As a nursing assistant, you are involved in nearly all communications in your nursing facility. But problems can come up. Often you need to communicate with people who have little time and even less patience. Sometimes you must work with those who can't seem to communicate clearly. Other times—and these may be the most difficult of all—you are asked to listen to an unhappy or angry person when there may be nothing you can do about it.

Most of us have no trouble communicating when things are peaceful and calm. But when we feel stressed, both listening well and speaking clearly are more difficult. But there's some good news: Anyone can learn to be a better communicator—really! Experts who have looked at nursing homes suggest some specific communication skills that work well in tense situations.

The first thing to do:

1st Improve your communication skills

Active listening

One of the best ways to improve your communication skills is to become an "active listener." When someone is talking, are you thinking of what you are going to say next? Or is your mind wandering to your next task? Make a conscious effort to stay focused on the person who is talking with you, and then think about how to respond.

Probably the most important part of being an active listener is to stay calm yourself. That lets you think about how the person you are talking to is feeling. Is the speaker frustrated, at the end of his or her rope? Is he or she upset? What is the real issue? Does the speaker want you to help solve a problem? Or is he or she just letting off steam?

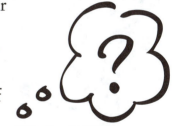

© Delmar/Cengage Learning 2013

We all need to express anger or complain from time to time. Trying to give specific suggestions when the other person really wants only sympathy can create misunderstanding and hurt feelings. On the other hand, offering only sympathy when the other person is looking for specific suggestions can be just as troubling.

So you need to listen well and carefully to the other person. That lets you know how to deal with him or her.

Feedback

An excellent communication tool is called "feedback." That is, after the other person is done talking, give a short summary of what you think has been said.

Sometimes it helps to give factual feedback, just so you and the other person are clear about what has been discussed or decided in a conversation. For example, after a discussion with a family member about a resident's clothing needs, you might say, "Okay, so you know that your mother needs some new housedresses, and you're going to bring them in next week. That sounds great." Both you and the family member will be more likely to remember that a decision has been made.

Feedback can also help with emotional issues. For example, if a resident's wife has described difficulties with her husband, you could say, "I understand that you feel bad about your husband's living here. It must be really hard." This makes the other person feel like she has been really listened to.

Have you ever had a conversation with someone where you felt they really didn't listen to you? You know, one that went something like this:

© Delmar/Cengage Learning 2013

Betty: *So that's the whole story. It looks like my husband is leaving me, and my daughter is flunking out of school, and the bank is going to take back my house.*

Marge: *Yeah. So what do you think of my new haircut?*

Okay, we know we're exaggerating here. But you know what we mean. It's so frustrating to feel like someone hasn't heard what you were saying. Giving feedback shows we've really listened to someone else, and we can overcome a lot of communication problems.

I-messages

Another simple but important tool is called an "I-message." This is particularly important in trying to resolve conflict. It is a good way to make sure you are saying what you mean without causing the other person to become angry or defensive.

For example, Corinna feels that Gwen is working too slowly and taking too many breaks, leaving her with more work to do.

Suppose she approaches Gwen like this: "You are so lazy! You always take a break any time you feel like it, and you always come back late. When you do work you're so slow that I end up having to do twice as much!"

The first thing Gwen heard was an accusation, or a "you-message." Most of us would get mad in a situation like this and stop listening. It is unlikely that Corinna will get her point across.

Now let's look at another approach Corinna might have taken using an I-message. The format of an I-message looks like this:

When _____ *happens,*

I feel _____

because _____.

I would like _____ *to happen.*

Here's what Corinna might have said, using an I-message: "Gwen, when you take extra time on your break, like you did yesterday, I feel frustrated, because it makes more work for the rest of us. I would like it if we could all get back from our breaks on time. That seems most fair to everybody. What do you think?"

Notice that Corinna did not judge Gwen as a person. She did not use the word *always*, and she did not blame her. Gwen may find it possible to put herself in Corinna's shoes, and that may help her to change her behavior. Notice also that Corinna seems to have waited a day, probably to calm herself, before speaking to Gwen.

The next step:

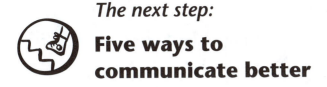

Five ways to communicate better

Try to make these good communication skills a daily habit. When you are having problems communicating with someone— a resident, a family member, a supervisor, or a coworker—try to keep these things in mind.

1. Invite discussion

Try asking "door opening" questions such as, "Want to talk about it?" or "You look upset. Is something bothering you?"

© Delmar/Cengage Learning 2013

1. invite discussion

2. empathize

3. be an active listener

4. avoid finger-pointing

5. avoid generalizing

2. Empathize

Try to put yourself in the place of the other person. Let the person know that you understand his or her situation. For example: "I'd like to hear more about your concerns," or "It must be difficult . . ."

3. Be an active listener

Try repeating what you have just heard. This can be comforting in itself. Say something like, "So, what you're concerned about is . . ."

4. Avoid finger-pointing

Blaming others is always a bad approach. "I-messages" are useful in keeping people from feeling blamed.

5. Avoid generalizing

The words *always* and *never* are rarely the right way to describe a situation, and they invite defensiveness.

Remember

When you have trouble communicating:

- **be sure you understand the real issue.**

- **provide feedback to be sure you've understood.**

- **use "I" messages.**

- **avoid blaming.**

- **do not generalize.**

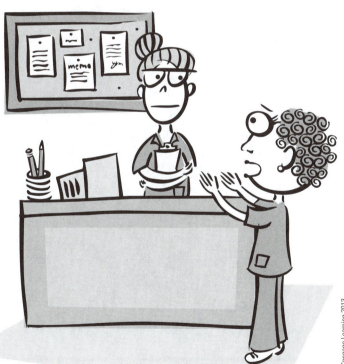

4

I need to get along with my supervisor?

As a nursing assistant, the law says you are a "dependent practitioner" in long-term care. In other words, you work under the direction of a licensed person—in your case, a nurse. Your relationship with your supervisor is important to your job satisfaction.

All good professional relationships are founded on respect. They also need clear expectations and good ongoing communication. These kinds of relationships take hard work and patience. The relationship between nursing assistant and supervisor is no exception.

The first thing to do:

Understand the CNA-supervisor relationship

Same goal, different role

You and your supervisor share a common goal—quality care for the residents of your facility. Your roles are different, however. It may be helpful to review your respective roles so that you have clear expectations, both for yourself and for your supervisor.

The role of the supervisor is a larger one than most nursing assistants see. The nurse's primary responsibility is to direct the care of the residents according to the orders prescribed by a physician. Depending on the size and organization of your facility, your supervisor may also be responsible for the following:

- Hiring new staff and finding replacement staff for absentees

- Training new nursing assistants and conducting in-service programs

- Preparing the facility for survey

- Notifying residents' families in the event of acute illness or death
- Coordinating the efforts of various specialists, such as PT/OT therapists, social workers, and psychologists

Your major role as a nursing assistant is to perform the daily hands-on care of the residents. It sounds simple until you understand what that little word *care* means. In addition to helping residents with activities of daily living, your role is to learn the residents' likes and dislikes and understand their family and cultural backgrounds and how these might affect their lives in the nursing facility. You help the resident to be more independent. You also work with residents' families and observe residents for any changes in their condition.

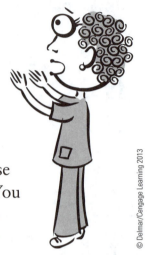

© Delmar/Cengage Learning 2013

In other words, you and your supervisor have something else in common: You are both extremely busy! Juggling so many tasks, trying to decide which is most important at any given time, responding to various demands from one moment to the next, creates stress, lots of it. Stress, in turn, makes communication both more important and more difficult.

Two-way communication

Being able to share information with your supervisor is essential to safety and quality of care. You depend on your supervisor's shift report for information about residents. Your supervisor depends on you to provide information about residents for the report to the next shift. This communication is basic, and no nursing unit can do without it. There are other kinds of communication besides these that are important to personalizing care, and to keeping a high morale.

Many nursing assistants feel that the only time they hear from their supervisors is when they've made a mistake. If you feel that this is true, try asking your supervisor for some time to discuss your strengths and weaknesses as a caregiver. Show your supervisor that you value constructive criticism. Ask for help with those parts of the job that you find most difficult. Take charge of your caregiving, and use your supervisor as a resource and a consultant.

respect

communication

teamwork

© Delmar/Cengage Learning 2013

It is normal to sometimes feel frustrated by the many communication breakdowns that can happen in a nursing facility. It is also easy to blame others. When nursing assistants blame the supervisor for problems and the supervisor blames the nursing assistants, communication stops.

The sharing of information is only part of good ongoing communication. Supervisor and nursing assistant are roles, but those roles are played by human beings who need encouragement, appreciation, and support. In other words, as a nursing assistant, you may need to reach out to your supervisor and begin to shape the kind of relationship you want and need.

Sometimes your troubles with your supervisor may be the result of a personality conflict between the two of you. In other words, you are continually "rubbing each other the wrong way." If you have always gotten along with supervisors in the past, and you are doing your best on the job, then you and your supervisor may be tangled in a conflict neither of you understand. In this case, it is important not to blame each other and to get help from someone who can assist both of you. A good person to talk to may be your facility's social worker.

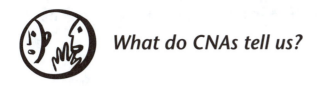 *What do CNAs tell us?*

We asked CNAs from around the country to tell us about how they work with their supervisors:

What is the most important advice you would give to other CNAs on how to get along with a supervisor?

SARA MUÑOZ

Benedictine Nursing Center, Mt. Angel, Oregon

"Be up front with them and keep the lines of communication open."

ROGER DINGESS

Westland Convalescent Center, Westland, Michigan

"Work together as a team. Don't bring your problems or moods from home to work with you. Be a friend and a coworker."

What is the best way to get off on a good foot with a new supervisor?

ROGER DINGESS

"Make yourself available to help them get to know the residents and staff. Be open with communication because you can probably learn something new from her. Do your job well."

What is the best thing a supervisor can do to help you do your job well?

CAROLYN WILLIAMS
Estes South, Birmingham, Alabama

"Say 'thank you' and let you know when you're doing a good job. Be encouraging."

JEN KEEFE
Golden View Health Care Center, Meredith, New Hampshire

"Be respectful of your opinions because you're the one giving most of the care."

ROGER DINGESS

"Keep you informed of changes in situation or in care of a resident. Communicate openly."

What do supervisors tell us?

And just to keep things fair, we asked some supervisors what they think about their relationship with CNAs.

What is the most important thing a CNA can do to help you?

SUE WIECZOREK

Director of Nursing, Villa Crest, Manchester, New Hampshire

"Communicate and have respect for each other's position. Keep each other updated of any new developments."

© Delmar/Cengage Learning 2013

What's the worst thing a CNA can do on the job?

FRENCHIE PIERCE
Director of Nursing, New Community Extended Care Facility, Newark, New Jersey

"Mutual respect is most important, so being rude to a supervisor, peer, or a resident is the worst thing."

How do you handle conflict with a CNA?

SUE WIECZOREK

"I make sure my door is open to them."

FRENCHIE PIERCE

"I let them know that they can always ask me questions and talk to me one-on-one with any problems they're having."

Remember

The dos of getting along with your supervisor.

DO:

- See your supervisor as a colleague and a resource.

- Ask for the information you need.

- Communicate information about changes in a resident's condition.

- Keep your sense of humor.

- Accept constructive criticism.

- Be flexible in accepting assignments.

- Ask questions if you are unsure what's expected of you.

Remember

The don'ts of getting along with your supervisor.

DON'T:

- See your supervisor merely as "the boss."

- Be reluctant or shy in seeking important information.

- Stop offering input about residents, even if you feel unheard.

- React to others' anger, irritability, or other stress-caused behavior.

- Take criticism of your work personally.

- Insist on certain assignments.

- Pretend to understand what you are in fact unsure of.

5

What do I do when . . .

I need to get along with family members?

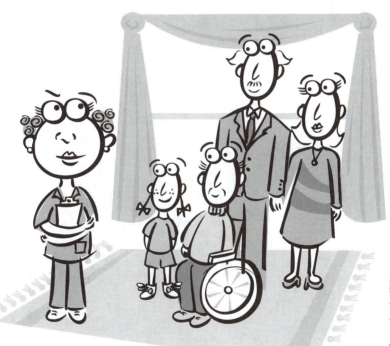

When nursing assistants and families work together, everyone benefits. Nursing assistants provide better care when families let them know about residents' special needs and problems. At the same time, families trust that their relatives are getting good care and residents have better quality of life and are happier.

The first thing to do:

1st Understand the importance of family members

Family members can ease the difficult transition to nursing home life. Their visits can help organize residents' time and add variety to their days. A short conversation between a relative and nursing assistant can also help the nursing home view someone as an excellent teacher or someone who loved to fish, not just as "an Alzheimer's resident."

However, communication gaps can cause trouble. Although family members can help residents in many ways, sometimes they confuse their roles with the nursing assistant's role. For example, husbands and wives of residents may still want to be the primary caregivers. At the same time, nursing assistants feel that they are responsible for care of the resident. Suddenly, tasks such as feeding or bathing a resident can cause conflict between relatives and nursing assistants.

© Delmar/Cengage Learning 2013

More conflicts can arise when families do not understand the nursing home environment. For instance, a relative might complain about things staff have to do because of state regulations. Or they may be upset about the resident's medications, which have been prescribed by her doctor. In cases like these, nursing assistants can take the blame for things they do not control.

Jane Traupmann, a family therapist who has worked in nursing homes, puts it this way:

> *Many families feel guilt about the decision to put their relative in a nursing home. They can feel both relieved and scared at the same time. The decision to place a loved one is almost always a very difficult one. It is helpful to nursing assistants if they can keep this in mind when they are having problems or conflicts with family members. Some of the anger families have about the whole situation may be directed at the nursing assistants, because they are the front line of contact for most relatives.*

The next step:

Some ways to get along better with family members

Express yourself

Just listening to a family's concerns can help you get along well with them. A sociologist who talked to more than 100 relatives of nursing home residents found that although family members were deeply concerned about quality of care, they were even more concerned about whether nursing assistants cared for their residents as people.

let me te you a little story about Dad...

It is easy to let family members know that you care. Try spending a little time talking with them when they visit your facility. Share with them your residents' daily activities, likes, and dislikes. This simple form of communication tells relatives that you are watching over their loved one and thinking of him or her not just as a resident, but as a member of the family.

© Delmar/Cengage Learning 2013

Sharing is also caring

Another way to help personalize resident care is by encouraging families to create a bulletin board (or scrapbook) with information about their loved one. The board can contain all kinds of things that let staff know about the history of the resident: photographs, awards, diplomas, letters—anything that highlights the resident as a person. This is a great way to share information about who the resident was before coming to the nursing home. It also offers important background for new staff who do not already know the resident, and it can serve as a conversation starter with families.

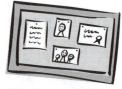

© Delmar/Cengage Learning 2013

Know your limitations

Remember that you do not have to do it all yourself. Sometimes family members will have persistent problems or complaints that you simply cannot fix. Make sure you report these difficulties to your supervisor, who can refer the family member to the social worker, director of nursing, medical director, or administrator. Remember that family members may not know to whom to speak about a problem, and pointing them in the right direction isn't "copping out," but instead can help get the problem solved.

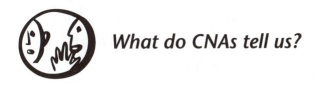

What do CNAs tell us?

Three CNAs shared their thoughts about relating to family members.

CAROL MCMANUS
Beverly Oak, Melbourne, Florida

"One resident today showed me some pictures of her grand-children that just came in the mail. I let her know how beautiful they are. She doesn't see too well, and I assured her that they looked very pretty. Then I told her about my own grandchildren. You have to remember that our families are important to all of us.

"I can't tell you any horror stories. I really enjoy the residents' families. They're all really nice. If you treat them with respect, then they respect you.

"I try to be like a friend. Talk with them about outside topics. I always treat them like a friend who's come to visit. My favorite part of this job is the interaction with the residents and their families.

"With new residents, it's all about letting the family know that you care about their family member; that the resident comes first; that you'll work hard to make their loved one feel like they're at home.

"I've had a few residents pass on. When their families come in to get their stuff, I try to treat them with respect, with empathy. I pack up the resident's stuff, so the family doesn't have to go through that.

"The worst thing you can do is disrespect the family."

DEBORAH DINWIDDIE
C. Davis Home, Wilmington, North Carolina

"When a new family gets here, they're usually real nervous. I make a point of getting right down there and introducing myself, with a big smile—you'd be surprised how people forget to do that. I make a point of letting them know they can always call me if they need anything.

"When a relative is angry or upset, I look them straight in the face and ask what's the matter, tell me about it, let's see if there's something we can do about it. Most people calm down quickly when they know someone is really listening."

SUSAN GOODWIN
Avalon Manor, Waukesha, Wisconsin

"Working with residents' families? It's the fun part of the job!

"I try to build real positive relationships. It's always on a first-name basis—it seems less formal, more homey. I personally like that.

"We need the family, because we need to know the resident. We need to find out what they like, and don't like. I enjoy talking to families; you can learn something about the resident that maybe you didn't know. It might come in handy later. We need to work together."

Remember

Always be sure to:

- Learn all you can from family members about the resident's life before coming to the nursing home.

- Let families know you care about their loved one, too.

- Help residents, family members, and staff communicate through bulletin boards, photo albums, and scrapbooks about the resident.

- Know your limitations.

- Use good communication skills with families.

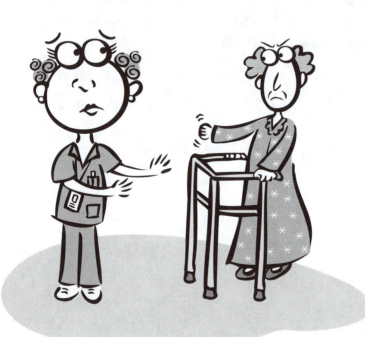

6

What do I do when . . .

Residents are angry and aggressive?

Dealing with verbal and physical aggression from residents is one of the most challenging parts of the nursing assistant's job. It's hard to know how to respond when residents become angry and yell or strike out at staff. In this chapter, we share some of the experts' ideas on how to understand and calm situations in which residents become aggressive.

The first thing to do:

1st Understand why residents get angry and aggressive

Hannah, a nursing assistant, brings a lunch tray to one of her residents. As Hannah tries to assist her, the resident yells out, "I'm sick and tired of being told what to do all the time—get

away from me!" The resident then hits Hannah and knocks the tray to the floor. Hannah feels like crying and wonders how the situation got so out of hand.

© Delmar/Cengage Learning 2013

Although we don't talk about it very often, this kind of situation is all too familiar to most nursing assistants. One large survey of nursing assistants found that most of them had been insulted or sworn at more than once in the past year. Further, many had been pushed, grabbed, or shoved by residents, or hurt in some other way at least a few times during the previous year. The nursing assistants found such incidents very upsetting, and they often felt powerless to prevent them.

Let's be honest: Of all the things that cause stress for nursing assistants, having angry confrontations with residents is just about the worst. Although you know that the resident is not doing it on purpose, you may get angry in return. And the part that's hardest is not knowing what to do. A nursing assistant who has just been hit or cursed at asks himself or herself: 'What could I have done? Was this my fault?'

X@!#GRRR!

© Delmar/Cengage Learning 2013

The first step in relating to aggressive residents is to understand why the behaviors occur. There are a number of major reasons, including:

- **Physical conditions**

  Injury to the brain can sometimes cause aggressive behavior. Dementia can also lead to verbal and physical outbursts, particularly among people with moderate levels of mental impairment. Many CNAs find that the most helpful thing they can do when a resident strikes out at them is to remember this fact: The person is doing it because of an illness that affects his or her behavior, not because he or she is "trying to be mean" or is a bad or nasty person.

- **Life experiences**

  Individuals with a history of violent behavior may be among your residents. These people may have dealt with anger by being aggressive or violent throughout their lives, and simply continue this behavior in the nursing home.

- **Environmental factors**

  When a resident feels out of control or frustrated with his or her immediate situation, he or she may strike out or yell at the caregiver. Because direct care situations such as bathing, feeding, and dressing can be confusing and frustrating for residents, aggressive behavior is likely to occur when direct care is being given.

© Delmar/Cengage Learning 2013

Understanding vs. taking things personally

An expert on aggression by residents, Beth Hudson Keller, suggests that nursing assistants try to avoid taking resident aggression personally. Unless you have done something to directly provoke a resident, you should remember that you are not personally responsible for the anger he or she feels. Beth also points out that all nursing assistants experience verbal or physical aggression from residents at one time or another, so it is not just your problem. To help residents and nursing assistants minimize aggressive behavior, staff need to work together to find the causes of the behavior.

© Delmar/Cengage Learning 2013

Concentrate on the Person

Perhaps the most helpful thing you can do is find out why the resident is angry, agitated, or combative. This may take some time, but understanding why the resident is angry or upset, rather than just trying to figure out how to complete a caregiving task, is worthwhile in the long run.

A concept called *person-centered care* is being used in more nursing homes. It is an active approach to thinking about and responding to residents in a new way. The behavior of a resident with dementia may seem strange and unpredictable to you, but the resident's behavior is an attempt to communicate a need, wish, or feeling. You need to look for the *meaning* behind the behavior.

The person-centered approach leads us to rethink our ideas about what are sometimes called "problem behaviors." By making a thoughtful attempt to understand the meaning behind a behavior, we can come up with new and more effective caring interventions.

Let's take the example of a resident who is sitting in the hallway, screaming continually. Both staff and other residents are becoming irritated, and the resident herself is clearly unhappy. How would a person-centered approach respond to this situation?

First, keeping in mind that behaviors have meaning, staff can assess why this could be happening. Knowing the resident as well as possible, what activity would be meaningful for the resident and redirect the resident? Is the resident expressing a need for sensory stimulation? How can these needs be met? Gentle massage? Giving the resident a textured blanket or stuffed animal? Does she need to be helped to the toilet, or is she hungry or thirsty? Bored? Is she in pain or discomfort? (What chronic illnesses does the resident suffer from that are associated with chronic pain?) By observing the resident and seeing how she responds to these kinds of interventions, the underlying need that stimulates the behavior can be identified.

This is what the person-centered approach adds to your caregiving toolkit. The behaviors of residents, and especially persons with dementia, must be looked at in fresh, new ways. As a CNA you can help immensely if you help look for the meaning behind residents' behaviors and work with other staff to come up with creative solutions.

When talking fails

Sometimes you will be able to talk about a situation with an angry resident and find a solution. However, especially when an aggressive resident has dementia, verbal communication may not give you information that helps you resolve the situation. Physical cues can be helpful in such cases.

Experts point out that it is important to approach the aggressive person calmly. If you carefully observe your residents, you can learn their individual signs of anger and frustration.

One way to calm an agitated resident is to sit down with him or her, spending a few quiet moments before you begin a caregiving task. This is especially important if the resident is already agitated. The key is to invest enough time in the situation to either calm the resident down or to make the environment feel calmer and safer.

If you feel you are getting angry yourself, take a few deep breaths, take a step or two backward, and ask yourself what is going on: "Okay, do I really have to do this now? Can I get somebody to help me? Can I come back later to do this task?" (One of the relaxation exercises we mentioned in Chapter 1 can help here.)

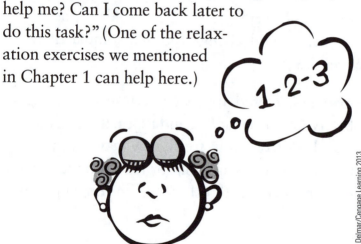

© Delmar/Cengage Learning 2013

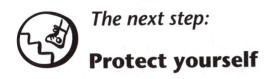

The next step:

Protect yourself

We can't eliminate all resident anger. But you can keep yourself from being hurt or injured by an aggressive resident. You need to know how to keep an angry situation from becoming an aggressive one. The following five tips may help.

1. Voice tone and volume

When a resident is yelling and shouting, shouting back will only aggravate the situation. Use a calm, nonthreatening tone.

2. Body posture

When someone is angry, we naturally want to place a reassuring hand on that person. However, this may lead to a negative physical response from the resident. He or she may interpret the gesture as an attack, even though it was not meant as one. It is important not to touch a resident when he or she is very angry. Also, be aware of your own posture toward the resident. Pointing one's finger or stiffening up will not help an angry resident. Make sure you are on eye level with the resident. If the resident is in a wheelchair, try to sit down next to him or her.

3. Distance

Stepping too close to a resident may make the situation worse. Moving too close may threaten the resident and make him or her strike out at you. Always give an angry person the room he or she seems to want.

4. Flexibility

If a resident is angry about a caregiving task you are trying to perform, stop the task and give him or her time to cool off. Remember, resident anger is often in response to a loss of control. Try to return a sense of control to the resident by offering to come back later or offering some options about how the task is done.

5. Get help

It is always a good idea to ask yourself if you are the best person to calm the aggressive resident. Perhaps the resident has a favorite staff person on whom you can call for help. Or you might find that you need some backup from a nurse or social worker to keep the situation manageable. It is best to ask for help if you need it.

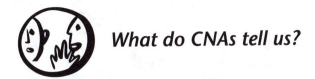 *What do CNAs tell us?*

Genevieve Gipson, designer of the Career Nurse Assistants Program in Ohio, asked nursing assistants about how they helped residents to feel calmer. Here are some of their ideas:

"Sometimes I've been scared residents were going to hit me or hurt me—but I stayed calm, and I believe it helped the residents stay calm."

"At the same time you are calming the resident down, you have to calm yourself also."

"Always, always tell them my name and call them by name."

"Never yell or startle a person."

"Be careful if they are daydreaming that I don't scare them."

"Give them time to answer before I go on."

"Pay attention to the little things and make small talk."

"Say exactly when I'll be back and then do it."

Remember

- Don't take resident aggression personally.

- Try to find out what upset the resident.

- Step backward or sit down with the resident.

- Speak in a calm, quiet voice.

- Come back later.

- Get help from other CNAs if necessary.

7

What do I do when . . .

My family and my job pull me in different directions?

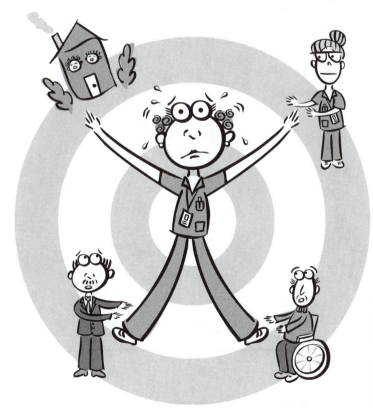

Often the best nursing assistants are those who already have some experience caring for others. However, for CNAs who parents of young children or who are taking care of aged parents, this means that you are never "off-duty." There never seems to be enough time. It feels like time itself is the enemy, and that someone either at home or at work is always being shortchanged. Knowing your limits can help you to better use your strengths in finding the right balance.

Take a look at family stress and how it affects you at work

Janet, a nursing assistant for six months, is a single mother of twin three-year-old boys and a five-year-old girl. Before deciding to work as a nursing assistant, she arranged for her mother to see her daughter off to kindergarten each morning and take care of the twins until she got home. Janet's mother was happy to have the time with her grandchildren, so this seemed like a perfect arrangement. Two weeks ago, however, Janet's mother suffered a stroke and was hospitalized.

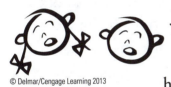

© Delmar/Cengage Learning 2013

Janet is afraid she will have to leave her job if she can't find child care. She also worries about her mother, who needs her help now. To top it all off, one of the residents recently complained that Janet was crabby and unfriendly.

No matter where she turns, Janet comes face to face with another demand. Some days she feels like a bad mother, a bad daughter, and, lately, a bad nursing assistant.

If you are a nursing assistant who also has family responsibilities, you are all too familiar with the stresses and strains of people like Janet. Learning to manage both time and stress can help you "balance the load." Especially when the problems seem overwhelming, you need to find a way to relax. When you are tense and worried, you can't sort things out and plan an effective strategy.

Nobody's perfect

Often caregivers, including nursing assistants, have high expectations of themselves. As long as these expectations are realistic, this kind of commitment helps us to be good caregivers both at home and on the job. But when our expectations for ourselves are too high, we tend to feel guilty for not meeting them, which creates stress.

When we are stressed we can't think clearly, and we make mistakes or exercise poor judgment. When we realize we have made a mistake, we feel guilty for that, too, which creates further stress, and on and on until we finally burn out.

If you are regularly feeling short-tempered and resentful, convinced that no matter how much you give of yourself no one appreciates you, you may be experiencing the beginning of burnout. Taking a good look at your expectations of yourself and making some adjustments is the first step toward balance.

Family therapists suggest that we give up the idea of being a "perfect mother" or "perfect father." The attempt to be a perfect parent is always doomed to fail. If a parent first decides which things are most important in being a good parent and finds ways to accomplish those, other problems are more easily solved; in fact, some of the other less important problems do not arise in the first place.

John Wood, writing in *Modern Maturity*, says that too many people think they must take care of their parents the same way their folks took care of them. Many studies show, however, that most older parents prefer to be as independent as possible. So we don't need to strive to be the "perfect family caregiver" either.

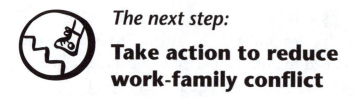

The next step:

Take action to reduce work-family conflict

Managing your time

Many of us use checklists to make sure we don't forget any of the things we plan to do. What's more important, however, is to rank the items on the list in order of priority.

Remember as well to schedule some time to enjoy a friend or an activity you like. To care for others, you have to refresh yourself. You can't keep pouring from the pitcher without returning to the well.

© Delmar/Cengage Learning 2013

Stress management

Look again at the chapter on stress in this book. Remember that one of the best ways to relieve stress is to take a few moments to breathe deeply, stretch, and relax the muscles of your back and legs. You can train yourself to do this whenever you are beginning to feel overwhelmed. Some people find that meditation, temporarily letting go of their worries, helps them to refresh themselves. Others train themselves to hum a favorite peaceful melody, no matter how jangled they might feel, until they feel calmer.

It is extremely important not to use medications or alcohol to reduce stress. Chemical "help" has costs that can include ill health, impaired judgment, and even addiction.

Reach out to other people

The most effective way to reduce stress is to talk with others who can help boost your morale, or who will just let you complain for awhile, or who can help you keep things in perspective. If you do not have a support group for nursing assistants in your facility, speak to your supervisor and consider organizing one. Stress levels go down when people are able to share their burdens.

As a nursing assistant, you work hard taking care of others. Sometimes the demands of work and family can seem to be pulling you in different directions. To find practical solutions, however, you have to stay calm, plan your time realistically, take care of yourself, and remember to ask others for help. If you are juggling the complex demands of being a nursing assistant with family responsibilities, then take a moment to give yourself a pat on the back. You deserve it.

Five tips to help "balance the load"

1. Know your own strengths and weaknesses

Everyone copes with some kinds of things better than others. Do not let pride prevent you from asking for help with situations that are especially hard for you.

2. Plan ahead

Try to anticipate the situations that really cause you stress, and have a plan ready. It is always better to plot strategy when you are not in the middle of a stressful situation.

3. Take mental and emotional "breaks"

Sometimes, going from one stressful set of demands to another, we get so "keyed up" that we can lose sight of the larger picture and forget what's important. Sometimes it is best to put the emotional burden of the situation down for a few moments.

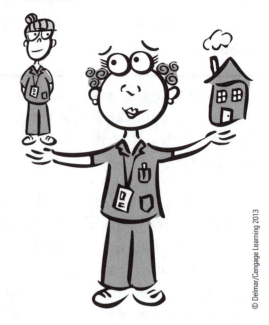

© Delmar/Cengage Learning 2013

4. Make definite transitions

Some people use the commute to and from work as a good time to empty themselves of stress. Clearly, bringing home the stress of the job isn't good for family relations. Neither is bringing the stress of family problems to work. Some people mark the transition with a ritual of some kind: taking your work shoes off at the door, for example (and leaving the work-day's stress behind with them when you cross the threshold). Others take off their CNA pin at the end of their shift and put it back on when they begin the next day to remind them of their professional identity.

5. Learn about local resources

Be sure to find out about the kinds of resources and services that are available in your community. There may be low-cost child care or subsidies to help you cover child care costs. If transportation is a problem, some communities have programs to help you secure a reliable car or get yours fixed. You can check out listings in your telephone directory for family and children's services, an office for the aging, and other helpful sources. Non-profit organizations where you live may also be able to help relieve work/family stress. Spend some time looking at what is offered in your city or town—you may be surprised at the help available!

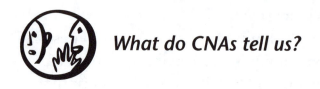

What do CNAs tell us?

We asked two CNAs who have family responsibilities how they manage the balancing act.

GWENDOLYN GOSA
Sunset Manor, Guin, Alabama
Three boys: Matthew (6), Tyler (5), Jon-Michael (1), and husband,
Christopher

"I work 7 to 3. My kids are in daycare. When I get home, I do my next job: taking care of the kids. It's hard. You just have to balance it out. I bathe them and cook supper. After I get them to bed I relax a little. Usually I'll take a hot shower, watch some TV, and then go to bed. I try to do soothing things.

"My husband helps me out a lot. He also works during the day—from 7:30 to 6 or 7 o'clock at night. He helps me not get so stressed out.

"I work weekends too. On weekends it's a little easier on me because my husband is off and can usually take care of the kids. He helps me more on the weekends than he can during the week."

Tips for new nursing assistants: *"Keep your calm, try not to get upset. It will come around. You have to pray a little bit too. Just have it in your head that you can do it, and be strong."*

CHRISTA CULVER

St. Vincent's Care Center, Bismarck, North Dakota

Two daughters: Jennifer (7), Kristi (6), and husband, Scott

"When my daughters were younger, I had quite a bit of help from my husband. We worked alternate shifts. I worked afternoon shifts, and we'd sort of swap in-between time at home with the kids. Now the kids are in school during the day. My husband brings them to school on his way to work, and I pick them up from school when I get done working at 2:30.

"My husband usually has Sundays off, but my schedule rotates. Sometimes it's just him and the girls. Sometimes it's just me and the girls. I like reading to them. Or one of them reads to me. I like to sit and listen to their stories.

"My husband and I are on a dart team together. So we set aside Wednesday nights for ourselves, and the girls go to grandma's house. That way we get some quality time as a couple.

"I actually think being a nursing assistant has helped my home life. At times you have to be real patient with residents, and that helps me be more patient at home, when the girls are fighting over something. Instead of taking one side, you try to hear both."

Tips for new nursing assistants: *"Value the days off with your kids. When it's wintertime, have snowball fights. Do little things, walk in the park or go to the zoo. Spend quality time with them."*

Remember

- First understand what competing demands are causing the conflict.

- Avoid the desire to be perfect in every area of your life.

- Manage your time.

- Manage your stress.

- Reach out to others for help and suggestions.

- Know your limits.

What do I do when . . .

I need to lift my spirits?

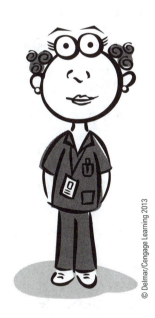

ost CNAs enjoy their work in the nursing home and find it very rewarding. But it's also the case that work life can sometimes get us down. We can have difficult conversations with coworkers, residents, or families. We can feel overworked, or problems in our personal lives might make us feel unhappy. Fortunately, there is a lot we can do to pick up our spirits and keep a positive attitude.

In fact, research shows that a positive attitude can lead to greater productivity at work and can help us stay healthy and happy. Our thoughts—positive or negative—affect the way we view the world and how others respond to us. Learning to channel them in a more positive direction can improve our interactions with others and lead to a more satisfying personal and professional life.

In his book *The Power of Positive Thinking*, Norman Vincent Peale wrote about a friend who carried a business card with this message: "The way to happiness: keep your heart free of hate, your mind from worry. Live simply, expect little, give much. Fill your life with love. Scatter sunshine. Forget self, think of others. Do as you would be done by. Try this for a week and you will be surprised."As a CNA, you have an opportunity to live out this message as you work with residents each day.

The first thing to do:

Be a positive thinker

We can all benefit from taking a look at our attitudes and how we present ourselves to others. Here are a few questions that may help you decide if it's time for an "attitude tune-up":

- Do you feel good about your work and personal life? Or do you dread certain aspects of your daily life, such as going to work?

- Do you usually expect a positive outcome or do you often fear that the worst will happen?

- Are you excited and energized by challenges, or do you feel overwhelmed and anticipate defeat?

- Do you often overreact to minor annoyances and criticism while ignoring or minimizing daily successes and compliments?

- Do you surround yourself with people of good humor, or are you drawn to those who constantly gripe?

If your answers reveal a trend toward negativity, it may be time to begin the journey to more positive thinking.

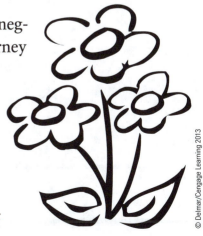

To practice positive thinking, we need to learn to pay attention to our "automatic thoughts." These are thoughts that trigger emotions in response to some situation or interaction. We are usually not aware of

© Delmar/Cengage Learning 2013

them because they happen so quickly. When automatic thoughts are negative, they get in the way of positive thinking and finding constructive solutions.

Here is a good way to tune in to your own automatic thoughts. Try to recall a recent irritating or frustrating event. Imagine it in slow motion and make a list of all the thoughts that run through your head as the situation unfolds in your mind. Now review your list and see if you can restate these thoughts more positively and realistically. For example, instead of thinking "Not another interruption! I can't get anything done!" substitute the equally valid thought, "Interruptions are to be expected. I usually get things done, and I can always get help if I need it."

With practice, you will learn to recognize your automatic thoughts as they occur and to replace them with more positive "self-talk."

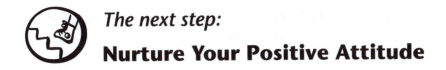

The next step:

Nurture Your Positive Attitude

Practice ways to calm down

Learning to quiet your mind with some form of silent meditation or prayer can be helpful. Think of it as a "mental vacation" that you can take whenever you have ten minutes to spare. Find a quiet a place (or use earplugs) and get in a comfortable position. Breathe slowly and deeply, concentrating on each breath in and out. Each time you find yourself thinking of a past or future event—a recent conversation, a chore you need to do—simply notice that your mind has strayed, then gently bring your attention back to your breathing. With practice, many people say that this form of meditation allows them to enter a peaceful state of mind at a moment's notice, often when they need it the most. Some find it difficult to clear the mind with silence and are more successful using music or chanting, which diverts the mind from conscious thought.

Practice self-acceptance

An important step in the journey to positive thinking is to believe in your self-worth. Recognize that you are unique, and challenge yourself to succeed by setting achievable goals.

Celebrate your daily successes with a gold star on your calendar, a small gift to yourself, or a mental pat on the back. Consider your mistakes a learning experience and a reminder that you are, after all, only human. Resist the temptation to judge yourself against others who appear more successful or competent. Take specific action to get the knowledge you need to feel competent. Consult a more experienced coworker or supervisor, take classes, read books and journals.

Practice proper perspective

It is easy to overreact to a negative situation when it has our full attention. To maintain perspective, slow down your automatic thoughts and reactions. When an unpleasant event or encounter happens, pause a moment, take a deep breath, and consciously choose how to respond. Ask yourself, "Is this really a big deal or just another bump in the road?"

In his book *First Things First*, Stephen Covey calls this "the moment of choice," and it is the essence of positive thinking. If someone is irritable and rude, you can still choose to remain cheerful and civil. Your choices at moments like these can make the difference between anger and frustration or a sense of peace and fulfillment.

Practice gratitude

When faced with major challenges such as illness or death, it is easy to allow negative thoughts to fill our minds. Try to focus on the "bigger picture," remembering what is still good in your life. It may help to write down all the positive aspects of your life and to express gratitude for them in a way that is meaningful to you.

© Delmar/Cengage Learning 2013

Reap the benefits

According to experts, positive thinking is good for your health. Research suggests that optimistic people recover more easily from heart attacks, back pain, and surgery. In one study, injured workers who practiced positive thinking recovered faster and returned to normal activities sooner than those who didn't.

Positive thinking is contagious. People are more likely to cooperate with someone who approaches them with a smile and an upbeat message. A coach is unlikely to inspire his team by saying, "There's a good chance we'll lose this game. Just do the best you can." A much more effective message would be, "We're up against a tough team, but so are they! Go out there and give it all you've got!"

As a CNA, you are in a position to make life better for the residents you care for each day. This is a tremendous contribution, not only to the individual residents but also to their families and everyone who cares about them. Whether you have chosen direct caregiving as a long-term career or a steppingstone to another endeavor, don't underestimate the impact your positive attitude can have on those around you. Stay positive whenever possible, for their sake and yours.

Finally, one important point: If after trying these techniques the idea of positive thinking seems impossible to you, you could be experiencing depression, a treatable illness. Some signs of depression are persistent feelings of sadness, hopelessness, worthlessness, difficulty sleeping, weight loss or gain, fatigue, lack of interest in activities that were once enjoyable, or thoughts of death or suicide. If that description matches how you are feeling, seek professional assistance so you can get the help you need.

Remember

- Scientific evidence shows that a positive attitude helps you handle stress, feel better, and stay healthy.

- You can take conscious steps every day to maintain a positive attitude.

- Be aware of negative "automatic thoughts" that can lower your mood.

- Practice using techniques such as gratitude, self-acceptance, and keeping things in perspective.

- If you find that negative feelings and a depressed mood are really getting you down, don't hesitate to seek the help of a counselor or other professional.

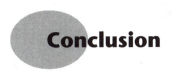

Conclusion

Your role is changing

As a nursing assistant, your role is changing. CNAs are now widely acknowledged as the primary caregivers in nursing homes—not just assistants to nurses. You are a valued member of the long-term care community, and your facility depends on you—on your skills, knowledge, compassion, and personal integrity.

You are directly responsible for the daily care and quality of life of the resident. You are the person in the facility who knows the individual resident's needs, wishes, hopes, fears, abilities. You are the one who can note subtle changes in mood, behavior, appetite, and general condition that may signal the need for tests or treatments by other members of the team.

You have a job to do that is different from anyone else's. You are a skilled, knowledgeable caregiver. But you are also a companion, friend, and ally. The tools of your trade are patience, empathy, and kindness. New buildings, fancy equipment, miracle medicines—none of these are as important to the quality of residents' lives as the loving care you provide on a daily basis.

Realize your worth

In a society that tends to rank people in importance according to the amount of money they make, it can be hard for you, as a nursing assistant, to realize your own worth. There probably aren't a lot of people lined up to thank you for the difficult and essential work you do. Many of the residents in your care are unable to thank you. Sometimes nurses and administrators become too busy with their own work to remember to express their gratitude. Too often families do not acknowledge your efforts. As a result, you can sometimes feel like the "low person on the totem pole."

Some CNAs have reacted to this feeling by adopting an attitude of "I just keep quiet and do as I'm told." In today's long-term care facility, however, you cannot be an effective caregiver with that attitude. Here's another way to look at it:

> *It's true that we're at the bottom, but that's not bad, that's good—we're the foundation! You don't build a house from the top down, you build it from the bottom up.*
>
> **—Ernestine Cofield, CNA**

In our work with CNAs over many years, in many different kinds of facilities, we have learned that it takes a special person to do this work. Not everybody is cut out for it. It takes courage, compassion, and creativity. And we also learned that all successful CNAs share a secret source of wisdom.

Thanks to you

Before we tell you that secret, however, there is something else we would like to say to you: Thank you. Thank you on behalf of your residents, their families, your employer, and your community for the care you give to the most vulnerable among us.

But thank you also for serving as a reminder of what is important in life. Turn on the television, or go to the movies and you might think that life is mostly about amassing fortunes, winning victories, or blowing things up. In the work you perform every day, however, you affirm the real meaning of what it means to be civilized, to be kind, to be human. So thank you for maintaining our hope and preserving our faith in people. Thank you for doing your best at being the best of us.

Now for the secret

Here is what we found out by talking to thousands of nursing assistants about their work. Are you ready? Here it is: They do it out of love. That's right. Love.

Think about it. People who do this work out of mere economic necessity do not last. Not in today's nursing home. Besides, there are a thousand easier ways to make a living.

Think about it some more. For a hundred dollars an hour, for a thousand dollars an hour, for any amount of money at all—could a person be a good nursing assistant, especially in some of the daily situations we've covered in this book, if they were not driven by love for other people?

But don't take our word for it. Listen to some of your colleagues:

> *I believe I'm working my way to heaven, just by doing my job. I've been a CNA for nearly 10 years now, and I wouldn't trade my profession for any other. No other job touches another's heart like being a CNA.*
>
> **—Becky Etienne, CNA**

You have to be a special person to be a nursing assistant. You have to be kind, caring, unselfish—we're professionals in our field. It really is a very rewarding career. You have to care about these people.

—Janet Desroches, CNA

This job is very rewarding if you think about it. I worked for 20 years as a Nurse Aide. Then I went back to school and became a Certified Nursing Assistant. I've always enjoyed it. You feel good, knowing they count so much on you. They're almost family. I love them.

—Elsie Tisdale Davis, CNA

We hope that you've found this book encouraging and useful. We hope that you'll refer to it when you're in tough situations, and we hope that you'll share what you've learned here with other CNAs.

And we hope you will never forget the value and importance of the work you do.

❖　❖　❖

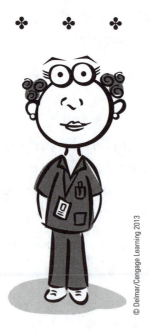